WITHDRAWN

Bilingual Edition
Let's Get Moving™
Edición Bilingüe

The JUMPING Book

SALTAR

Maya Glass

Traducción al español:
María Cristina Brusca

The Rosen Publishing Group's
PowerStart Press™ & **Editorial Buenas Letras**™
New York

Published in 2004 by The Rosen Publishing Group, Inc.
29 East 21st Street, New York, NY 10010

First Edition

Developmental Editor: Nancy Allison, Certified Movement Analyst, Registered Movement Educator
Book Design: Maria Melendez

Photo Credits: All photos by Maura B. McConnell.

Glass, Maya
The jumping book = Saltar / Maya Glass ; translated by María Cristina Brusca.
    p. cm. — (Let's get moving)
Includes index.
Summary: Pictures and brief captions describe the movements involved in jumping.
ISBN 1-4042-7513-4 (lib.)
 1. Jumping—Juvenile literature   [1. Jumping   2. Spanish language materials—Bilingual]
I. Title II. Title: Saltar   III. Series
  QP310.J86 G56 2004
  573.7'9—dc21
                                                          2003-009046

Manufactured in the United States of America

Due to the changing nature of Internet links, PowerStart Press has developed an online list of Web sites related to the subject of this book. This site is updated regularly. Please use this link to access the list:

http://www.buenasletraslinks.com/lgmov/saltar/

Contents

Contenido

I jump.

Salto.

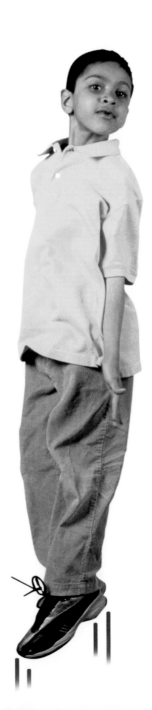

5

I jump high.

Salto muy alto.

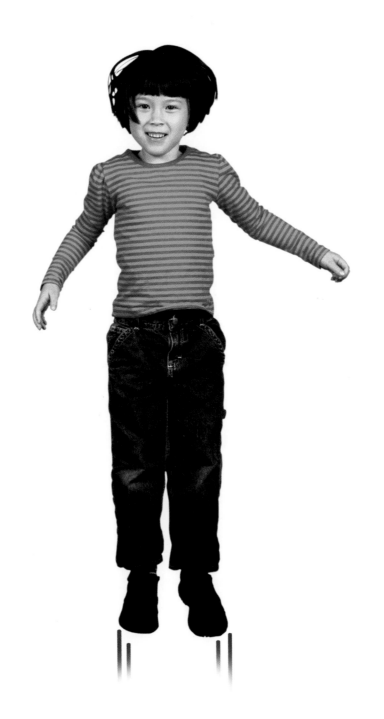

7

I jump higher.

Salto más alto.

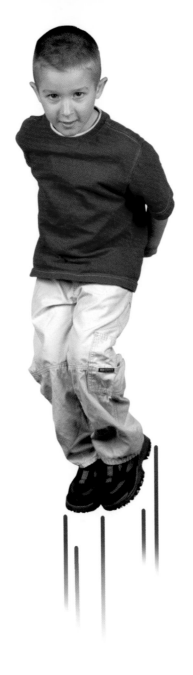

9

I jump up.

Salto hacia arriba.

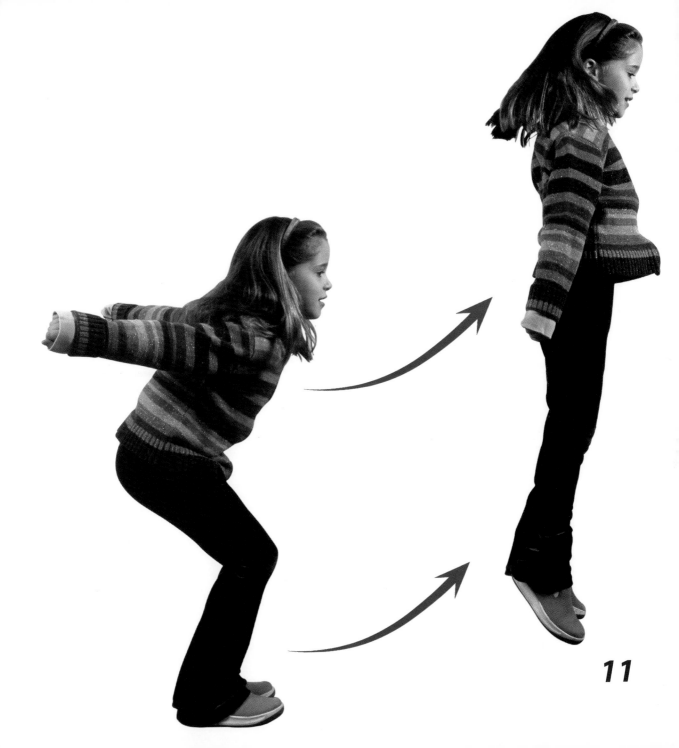

11

I jump down.

Salto hacia abajo.

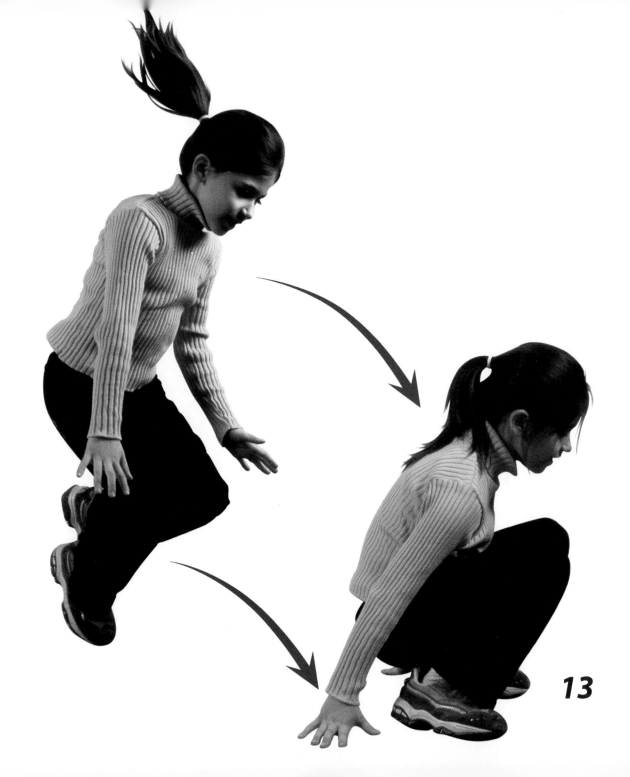

13

I jump
over here.

Salto por aquí.

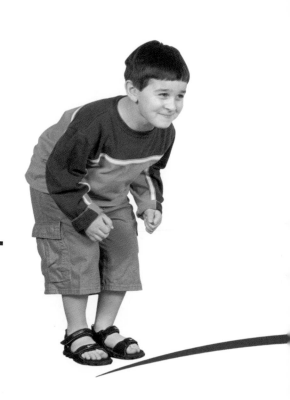

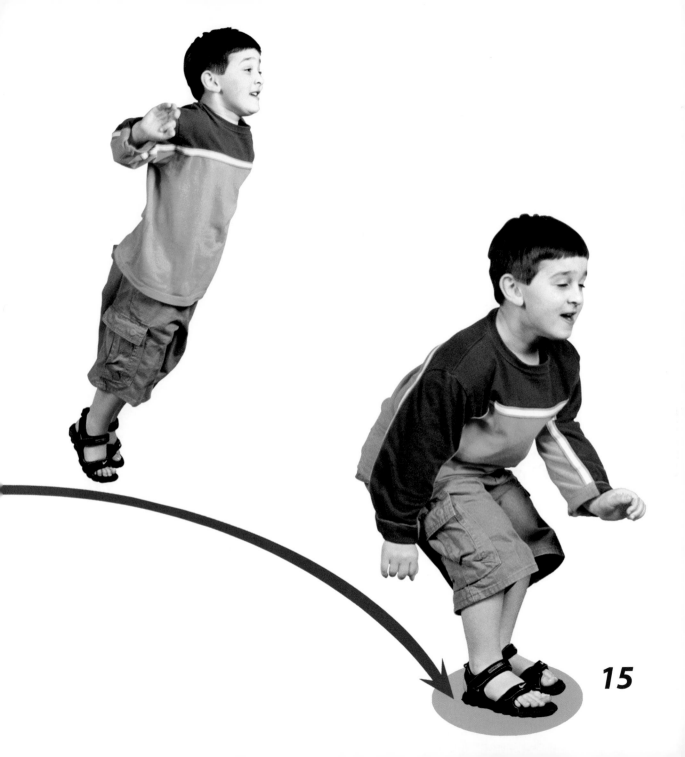

15

I jump
over there.

_____

Salto por allá.

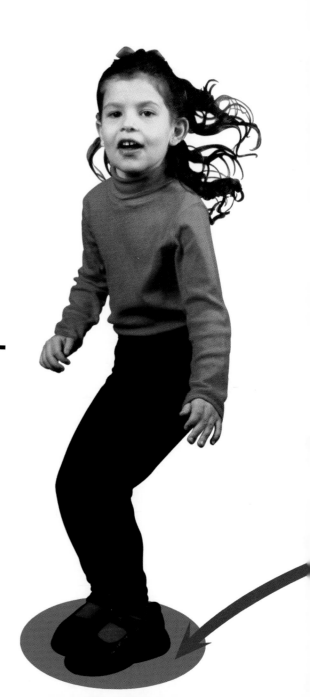

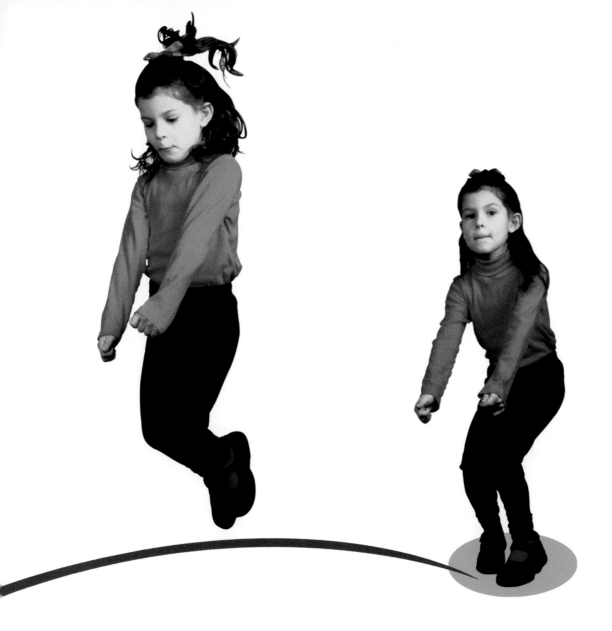

I jump with my arms
and legs together.

_____

Salto con las piernas y los
brazos pegados al cuerpo.

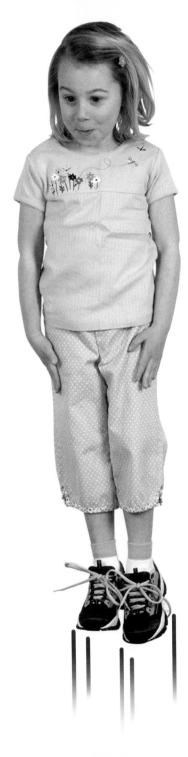

19

I jump with my arms
and legs apart.

Salto con las piernas y
los brazos abiertos.

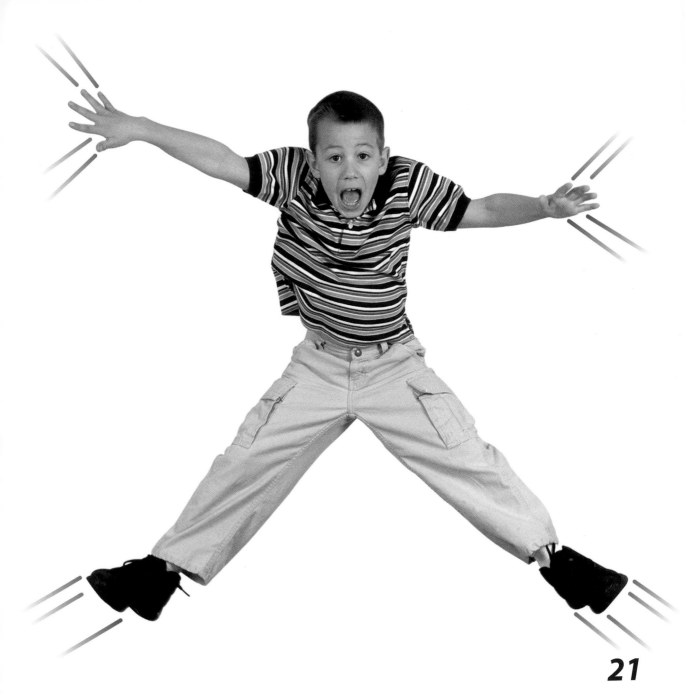

21

Jumping is fun!

¡Saltar es divertido!

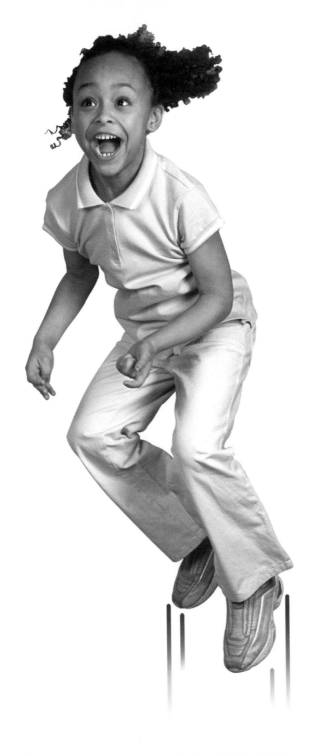

23

Words to Know
Palabras que debes saber

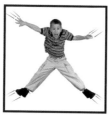

apart
abierto

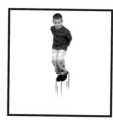

higher
más alto

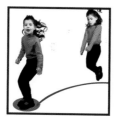

there
allá

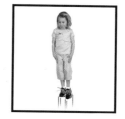

together
pegado